HOW TO PARENT TEENS WITH ANXIETY: Raising Calm And Confident Teens In An Anxious Generation.

Dorothy C. Jordan

Table of Content

INTRODUCTION:

It can be challenging to determine when ordinary teen stress turns into anxiety symptoms in adolescents. Teenagers with anxiety disorders, however, frequently experience significant levels of anxiety, and these emotions worsen over time rather than getting better on their own.

If anxiety is not treated, it can have a severe effect on a teen's ability to succeed in school and their relationships with friends and family. Adolescent anxiety can also result in co-occurring disorders including substance abuse and food disorders.

What Is Anxiety?

Anxiety is more than just worrying excessively. Worry is the act of obsessively thinking about problems, challenges, or

uncertainties—typically worries about the future or things we can't control.
However, anxiety is distinguished by unreasonably high levels of anxiety and distress that interfere with a teen's ability to operate properly.

It might be difficult to tell when typical teen stress evolves into anxiety symptoms. However, considerable levels of anxiety are regularly experienced by teenagers with anxiety disorders, and these feelings intensify over time instead of improving on their own.

Teenagers' ability to excel in school and their relationships with friends and family can suffer greatly if anxiety is not handled. Co-occurring disorders, such as substance misuse and eating disorders, can also be brought on by adolescent anxiety.

Chapter 1

A generation full of anxiety

Young people experience anxiety on a greater scale than earlier generations due to the rise of social media platforms and the general stresses of living in the digital age.

Anxiety in teens
Teen depression and social anxiety are just a few mental health disorders that appear to be the most common in the teenage cohort.

Mental health issues are widespread for young adults growing up in a world where technology has many of us glued to our phones instead of enjoying friendships in real-time

Youth anxiety
The prevalence of mental illness among teenagers and college students can be shown

in some major areas supported by the evidence.

Teenagers can avoid feeling their emotions by using technology like phones and laptops, which prevents them from developing resilience.
Teenage anxiety disorders are on the rise, which is a reflection of societal and cultural changes that have been noticed over the past few decades.

Due to biological variables and DNA, it is impossible to completely prevent juvenile anxiety problems, but more may be done to support adolescent anxiety management and promote mental toughness.
why there are more adolescents with anxiety than ever before
why there more adolescents with anxiety than ever before
Many young people, according to mental health practitioners, attend their clinics with

symptoms of panic disorder and anxiety disorder.

Research shows that anxiety among adolescents is widespread, with many psychotherapists saying that anxiety disorders are often the cause of why people of all ages, including teenagers, enter therapy.

Excessive worry
Some of the literature reported many reasons why anxiety disorders are so common among teenagers and young adults.

The reasons for anxiety disorders can vary, with many young people experiencing feelings of crippling failure and over-achievement.

Some teens worry so much about what their family and friends think they cannot function at all.

High anxiety levels
Many teenagers have endured challenging circumstances throughout their young lives, while others have functional, stable home environments with loving, supportive family members.

Cultural and societal changes
According to studies, high stress and anxiety among teens could be because of cultural and societal changes in recent decades.

Many teens feel pressure to do well and over-perform more than ever before and worry that they may not be on par with their peers.

Anxiety cluster
There is a difference between normal anxiety and the cluster of anxiety disorders: panic attacks, generalized anxiety disorder, social phobia, and obsessive-compulsive disorder.

Many people assume that anxiety is just a feeling of being nervous or on edge. While these symptoms are often present, anxiety disorders can cause many physical symptoms and mental health issues.

Other challenges
At times, anxiety makes us feel as though we are going crazy, and often, the symptoms can be so crippling that many people feel as though they might die, particularly in cases where someone has a panic attack.

Why do teens suffer from anxiety?
There are several reasons some of which get highlighted below

#1. Toxic happiness
Within our toxic positive culture, most kids and teens get taught that being happy all the time is acceptable, and unfortunately, many

parents think that it's their job to make sure that their child is happy twenty-four-seven.

All this is unrealistic and teaches children that other emotions such as anger, sadness, and frustration are unacceptable.

Feelings that remain suppressed often cause people to feel anxious and depressed.

Unfortunately, many kids grow up thinking that they have to be happy all the time, and if they're not, something must be wrong.

#2.Escaping through technology
Constant access to the internet and social media has presented many new challenges for teenagers growing up in the digital age.

Instead of addressing feelings of boredom, worry, and sadness, children pay attention to their screens and computer games.

Studies show that children over the millennia have gotten conditioned to avoid discomfort through the use of electronics.

Gaming and social media have replaced opportunities to build resilience and mental strength; thus, children haven't gained the coping skills required to handle everyday challenges.

#3. Not having enough free time to play
While attending sports clubs and other structured social events is critical, so is unstructured play.

Playtime without the confines of a club or teacher teaches children vital skills, such as managing conflict and disagreements without being guided by an adult.

In contrast, solitary play teaches kids how to be by themselves and comfortable in their skin.

#4. Giving children excessive praise
While it's essential for parents to encourage their children, too much praise often produces the opposite effect.

For example, when a parent tells their child "they are the best badminton player in the class" or that they are the most "intelligent in their school year", this often sets the precedent for excessive pressure where kids do their best to live up to the label.

The stress associated with "being the best" often produces profound fear of failure and rejection.

#5. Family dynamics are out of tune
As much as children and teenagers pretend to hate rules, deep down, they are well aware that they cannot always make the best decisions and require stable parental figures to guide them.

Children want their parents and caregivers to take the lead, even if they might not always agree or downright rebel against any rules put in place.

But, unfortunately, when the family dynamics are confusing or chaotic, a child's anxiety levels can go through the roof. Fortunately, anxiety disorders are highly treatable conditions.

When it comes to teen anxiety, it may be helpful for individuals to speak to a family member about how they are feeling.

Chapter 2

Into the mind of a teen

Pre-adulthood can be an extremely difficult stage, for your kid as well as for you too. Most guardians tragically feel that they realize what is happening inside the high school mind since they, at the end of the day, have had to deal with this. In any case, you need to understand that times change thus do the circumstances your kids face.

The way to successful nurturing is having comprehension. You want to realize what happens inside the high school mind. Not about their thought process, why their minds work how they do. Here is some knowledge that might end up being useful to you grasp your adolescent kid.

The sort of perspectives and thinking skills youngsters create at this age is vital to their change into adulthood. The high school mind is effectively affected so you must watch out. The following are a couple of focuses you ought to zero in on:

Attempt to cause your kids to understand the results. Teenagers are personal, so attempt to show them an obligation. Make them see the associations between their activities and the result through sensible thinking. They may not answer right away however they will ultimately learn.

Attempt to give them their space. Teenagers need to manage a ton of physical changes. Allow them to track down their own close-to-home outlet. Simply keep a check that it is a valuable thing.

The teen psyche will in general think just as far as the ongoing circumstance since they haven't created foreknowledge yet. This can cause sorrow and nervousness, particularly if they can't see past a disappointment or a terrible encounter. Assist them with the understanding that there will be a period past the present. Instruct them that terrible times will elapse and their feelings about the ongoing conditions will ultimately change.

Be patient and tune in. On the off chance that you attempt to make all the difference by taking a hold of your child's life, then they won't ever figure out how to make moves all alone. All things considered, assist your youngster with coming to the rt without help from anyone else. Attempt to be a thoughtful ear for them when they are in a difficult situation and be their aide.

Chapter 3

How can l identify anxiety in my teen?

To distinguish adolescent tension, getting more familiar with signs and symptoms is significant.
What's the distinction between indications of nervousness in youngsters versus side effects of uneasiness in adolescents?

Cautioning signs include conduct changes that can be seen by guardians, other relatives, educators, and companions. Side effects, then again, are a youngster's internal encounters, including intense subject matters along with actual grumblings, as they battle with nervousness.
That is the reason both perception and discussion are important to take a youngster's psychological wellness temperature.

The most effective way to recognize advance notice indications of uneasiness in teenagers is to notice your youngster's conduct consistently. Focus on their eating and resting propensities as well as their temperaments. Notice whether their regular exercises and communications have changed or decreased. Their presentation in school is likewise a telling mark of whether they might be experiencing uneasiness.

With regards to recognizing nervousness side effects in youngsters, and keeping up with them, open correspondence is urgent in figuring out your kid's perspective and interior experience, standard parent-kid correspondence can keep emotional wellness issues from grabbing hold or deteriorating. Research shows that side effects of nervousness in teenagers are more normal and more serious when youths' association with their folks has become more fragile. In this way, while chatting with a high schooler may not be simple, it merits the work.

Nervousness jumble side effects
There are numerous side effects related to uneasiness problems which can change as per the tension issue type. In any case, a portion of the advance notice indications of a tension problem include:

- Having a feeling of looming destruction or risk

- Feeling tense, anxious, or fretful.
- Fast relaxing
- Perspiring
- Feeling drained or frail.
- Resting issues
- Sensations of serious trepidation
- Chest torment
- Inconvenience concentrating
- Tight muscles
- Feeling restless or apprehensive, especially in friendly circumstances.
- Expanded pulse
- Experiencing issues controlling concerns where you frequently feel overpowered
- Having the desire to keep away from circumstances that trigger nervousness
- Substance misuse

Helping or hindering?

As a parent, you are the individual that your teen looks upward to. Be a good example by being a decent impact on them.

Your activities will inevitably impact your kids, so feel free to have a serious conversation regarding the outcomes of their activities. This will help them comprehend and answer in like manner to circumstances.

Remind your high schooler that they are solid and can do anything as long as they put their energy into it. Assist them with seeing that they are the ones who can lift themselves above awful circumstances.

Cause them to feel significant by showing real interest in the things they like. Pay attention to hip-bounce music assuming this they're into. Simply recollect that you don't need to like the class in the manner in which they do.

Continuously be available on occasion when they seem, by all accounts, to be disturbed. Some of the time, they just need a grown-up to pay attention to them.

Simply be cautious with your judgment. You maintain that your teenagers should see you as a protected spot where they can act naturally. Allow them to be powerless around you without faulting or fixing their concern for them. Additionally, be extremely aware of what guidance to give them.

Chapter 4

Natural ways of coping

At its root, uneasiness is a terrible reasoning propensity. The uplifting news? habits are conceivable! In Matthew 6:25-34, Jesus tells us not to be restless! He tells us not to stress over tomorrow, for it has the sufficient difficulty of its own, and to zero in on the day within reach.

The following are several methods for assisting our children with changing their restless reasoning propensities and leading them toward a better outlook by keeping them zeroed in on the present.

1. Establishing Procedures For Assisting Youngsters With Nervousness

It is vital to train them in the present. Tension spotlights on "imagine a scenario in which" rather than "what is." savvy to know about things that will occur from now on and get ready for them, however, this should be possible without nervousness. It is likewise fundamental for us to perceive conditions on the planet as unchangeable as far as we might be concerned in any case and let those things go.

For instance, Jane has a science test coming up on Friday. She can become restless about bombing the test or know about it and make sufficient arrangements for it by examining it. Those arrangements will take care of from here on out and it's something your youngster can do today.

At the point when your adolescent is feeling restless, go through the accompanying inquiries and have them answer the inquiries resoundingly if conceivable.

- Name five things that you can see at this moment.
- Name five sounds that you can hear at present. (Your adolescent can utter up sounds - like licking their lips, applauding, and so on, to additionally bring them back into the present.)

- Name five things that you can truly feel at present (like air from the fan, your fingers against the work area, and so on.)

When your youngster has addressed these three inquiries and named five things for each, pose them one final inquiry:

- What is the one thing I should think about or do at present?

The initial three inquiries in this strategy will assist with establishing your youngster in the present as opposed to from now on.

Pose the fourth inquiry once your high schooler has moved their concentration back to the present. This last inquiry is essential for educating the mind on where to go and how it will think pushing ahead.

Routine and Reiteration

It takes somewhere in the range of two to four months for our minds to untrain themselves from old reasoning examples and learn new ones. One basic method for achieving this is through daily practice and redundancy.

Redundancy reworks our cerebrum's brain processes and is how we advance as individuals. Hence, rehashing the above method can assist your teenagers with creating solid reasoning propensities.

Have your youngster do the 3×5+1 strategy no less than three times each day:

1) At the crack of dawn

2) At some point during the day (a mid-day break, for instance)

3) As they are preparing for bed.

It will require investment to lay out this everyday practice and to see the aftereffects of the work. Notwithstanding, as your adolescent continues to rehearse this everyday practice, genuine concerns will happen less and less habitually.

Tension can go crazy on the off chance that we're not being purposeful about retraining our cerebrums and guiding them by they way they ought to think. We should take "the changing of the brain" truly.

2. Guardians Assume a Part

Guardians, investigate yourselves and your tension levels. How frequently do you encounter nervousness? On the off chance that you battle with uneasiness, making the above strides with your children can be an extraordinary method for quieting the tension in yourself and assisting your children with conquering it. Practice the above strategies together. You'll find that it empowers you to beat feelings of apprehension as well as will help you and your high schooler bond too.

Center around the Present

Likewise, investigate what you might be deliberately or unwittingly imparting to your children. Recall that regardless of whether you mean something one way, your children might unexpectedly decipher your words. For instance, how frequently do you advise them to be protected or wear clean clothing in the event they're in a car crash?

Do you get some information about where they will head off to college, what their certificate plan will be, and the way that they will pay for it? Might it be said that you are pushing them toward greatness in their lives, or would you say you are empowering hairsplitting? Are your inquiries and guidelines future-zeroed in as opposed to what your youngster can do at this moment? While a portion of these discussions are indispensable to have and make arrangements for, how guardians convey them can increment nervousness.

Guardians can likewise exacerbate nervousness by permitting their youngsters' tension to turn into a huge concentration. A line between being merciful and supporting their tension. Continually yielding to it and pampering your youngster when they experience it will just aggravate it.

At the point when your teen is restless, rather than telling them, "It'll be OK," tell them, "You're alright at this moment. Gesture your head, let me know that is no joke." Regardless of whether they feign exacerbation, your adolescent has drawn in and returned to the present.

Be Thoughtful
Ensure your children realize that you love them for who they are on the right track now. Be certain they don't decipher your affection as something they can accomplish

just when they are less restless or "adequate."

Keep in mind, guardians, be generous with yourselves and your children. It's not difficult to become perfectionistic about being a parent and stress when things aren't going as well as you had trusted. Give yourself and your children the beauty to have those minutes, yet additionally to learn and develop.

Conclusion:
There is by all accounts a development of flawlessness and correlation, which causes uneasiness among youngsters instead of cultivating association and strength.

This can cause numerous emotional wellness issues for the youthful, receptive personalities of youngsters and teens.

It means a lot to help our children to live with a little distress and feel great trepidation by training them to do productive things to plan for what's to come. Laying out solid examples that assist them with beating that apprehension and uneasiness is one of the most amazing approaches to assisting adolescents with nervousness.

If you are prepared to acquire endless techniques to help your high schooler thrive in the present restless society?

Then, tap the "Add to Cart" button NOW